SIMPLIFIED

MEDICINE

DR MIRIAM KINAI

CONTENTS

DR MIRIAM KINAI

1

BILE DUCT CANCER

WHAT IS BILE DUCT CANCER?

Bile duct cancer, which is also known as cholangiocarcinoma, is a rare type of cancer which affects the bile ducts.

Bile is a liquid that is produced by the liver to help digest fats. This bile flows through bile ducts from the liver to the gall bladder where it is stored and to the small intestines where it used for fat digestion.

Bile ducts can be divided into two groups:

1. Extrahepatic ducts or the bile ducts that are outside the liver from which most bile duct cancers arise.

2. Intrahepatic ducts or the bile ducts inside the liver in which 5-10% of all cholangiocarcinomas develop.

***

WHAT CAUSES BILE DUCT CANCER?

The exact cause of most types of bile duct cancer is not known. However, risk factors which increase a person's chances of developing bile duct cancer include:

1. Having ulcerative colitis

This is an inflammatory condition which affects the intestines.

2. Having primary sclerosing cholangitis

This is an autoimmune disease in which the body's immune system attacks the bile ducts.

3. Having congenital bile duct abnormalities

Being born with choledochal cysts and other abnormalities of the bile duct system increases a person's risk of developing bile duct cancer.

4. Liver fluke infestation

Being infested by the liver fluke parasite which is common in Africa, Middle East and Asia is also thought to be another risk factor for bile duct cancer. A person becomes infested by eating undercooked fish that contains the parasite's eggs.

5. Exposure to chemicals

Being exposed to chemical in the rubber and automotive industries like dioxins, nitrosamines, and polychlorinated biphenyls (PCBs) can cause bile duct cancer to develop.

6. Advanced age

Most people who develop this cancer are usually more than 65 years.

7. Liver cirrhosis

Liver cirrhosis is a condition which can develop due to abusing alcohol and viral infections like hepatitis B and C.

WHAT ARE THE SYMPTOMS OF BILE DUCT CANCER?

Symptoms of bile duct cancer are caused by inability of the bile to flow from the liver where it is produced to the intestines where it is used since the tumor blocks the ducts.

As a result, the bile flows back into the bloodstream and the person develops jaundice. Jaundice is characterized by the whites of the eyes becoming yellow, the skin becoming yellowish and itchy, the urine developing a dark yellow color and the stool becoming whitish.

Other symptoms of cholangiocarcinoma include anorexia or loss of appetite, weight loss, vomiting, abdominal pain and fevers.

***

WHAT TESTS ARE DONE FOR BILE DUCT CANCER?

Investigations for patients with bile duct cancer include:

1. Liver function tests

These include bilirubin and alkaline phosphatase levels.

2. Tumor markers

Tumor markers that associated with bile duct cancer include carcinoembryonic antigen (CEA) and CA 19-9.

Having high levels of these tumor markers does not mean that a person has bile duct cancer since they can be caused by other diseases. In addition, persons with bile duct cancer may have normal levels of these markers.

3. Ultrasound scan

An ultrasound of the bile ducts, liver and other surrounding organs is done to evaluate the extent of the tumor.

4. CT (computerized tomography) scan

A CT scan of the abdomen uses x-rays to take pictures that give more details about the extent of the tumor.

5. MRI (magnetic resonance imaging) scan

A MRI scan uses magnetism to take pictures that give more details about the extent of the tumor.

6. ERCP (endoscopic retrograde cholangio-pancreatography)

In this procedure the doctor passes a small tube with a tiny camera into the small intestines and injects a dye into the bile ducts. This dye helps to take pictures of the bile ducts to determine if there are any abnormalities or blockages. If a blockage is found, it can be unblocked by passing a stent into the duct. The doctor can also take a biopsy or a small piece of tissue to be examined under the microscope for the presence of tumor cells.

5. PTC (percutaneous transhepatic cholangiography)

In this procedure the doctor passes a needle through the skin into the liver and injects dye into the bile ducts. This dye helps to take pictures of the bile ducts to see if they are abnormal or blocked. The doctor can also take a biopsy or a small piece of tissue to be examined under the microscope.

6. Angiogram

In this procedure a dye is injected into a blood vessel and x-rays done to see whether the cancer has spread into them from the bile ducts.

7. Biopsy

In this procedure a small piece of tissue is taken from the bile duct and examined under the microscope to confirm the presence of tumor cells.

8. Laparatomy

This procedure is done while the patient is under general anesthesia and the doctor makes a cut into the abdomen to examine the bile ducts for cancer. If it is found, the doctor removes it.

***

WHAT IS THE TREATMENT FOR BILE DUCT CANCER?

The treatment of bile duct cancer depends on the size of the tumor, its location and whether it has spread outside the bile duct. This treatment includes:

1. Surgery

This is done under general anesthesia and if the cancer is at a very early stage, only the affected bile ducts are removed.

If it has spread to the liver, then the affected parts are also removed (partial liver resection).

If the cancer has spread to other organs like the stomach, small intestines, pancreas, gall bladder and lymph nodes, these are removed in an operation known as Whipple's procedure.

2. Stent Insertion

If it is not possible to remove the tumor surgically, the surgeon can insert stents into the blocked tubes to relieve the obstruction.

3. Radiotherapy

High energy rays are used to destroy the cancer cells and shrink the tumor when it is not possible to remove it surgically.

This can be done by using an external radiotherapy machine or by placing radioactive material inside the body near to the tumor.

4. Chemotherapy

Cytotoxic or anti-cancer drugs are given to destroy the cancer cells if the entire tumor cannot be removed by surgery or the tumor recurs after initial treatment.

5. Chemoradiation

This is a combination of chemotherapy and radiation which is given to patients after surgery or to those patients who cannot have the tumor removed surgically.

WHAT IS THE PROGNOSIS FOR BILE DUCT CANCER?

The five year survival rate for early extrahepatic cancer is 30% and 15% for early intrahepatic cancer.

This means that 30% of people diagnosed with early extrahepatic cancer (cancer affecting bile ducts outside the liver) live for five or more years while 15% of people diagnosed with early intrahepatic cancer (cancer affecting bile ducts inside the liver) live for five or more years.

*****

2

OSTEOSARCOMA

WHAT IS OSTEOSARCOMA?

Osteosarcoma is a type of cancer that affects bones.

The most commonly affected bones are the:

1. Tibia (shin bone)

2. Femur (thigh bone)

3. Humerus (upper arm bone)

Other bones that are affected include the ribs, shoulder, spine, skull and pelvic bones.

***

WHAT CAUSES OSTEOSARCOMA?

The exact cause of Osteosarcoma is not known.

***

WHO GETS OSTEOSARCOMA?

Risk factors for developing Osteosarcoma include:

1. Adolescence

Osteosarcoma usually affects teenagers aged around 15 years during periods of rapid bone growth. It usually develops from the cells called osteoblasts which make the bone. Boys are more commonly affected than girls.

2. Being tall

Being tall for a certain age is thought to be one of the risk factors

3. Radiation treatment

Having received radiation treatment at a young age for cancer is also thought to be another of the risk factors.

4. Retinoblastoma

This cancer of the retina inside the eye can be part of a cancer syndrome that also includes osteosarcomas.

5. Li-Fraumeni syndrome

This is a genetic mutation (gene change) that is inherited and is associated with many cancers like brain, bone, soft tissue and breast cancers.

***

WHAT ARE THE SYMPTOMS OF OSTEOSARCOMA?

Symptoms of Osteosarcoma include:

1. Fractures of the bone

2. Pain in the bone. This can be worse at night or during exercise.

3. Pain when using the limb

4. Reduced range of movement

5. Swelling and redness on the affected leg or arm

6. Limping

***

WHAT TESTS ARE DONE FOR OSTEOSARCOMA?

Investigations for patients with Osteosarcoma include:

1. Blood tests like a full blood count to check the blood level.

2. X-ray

An x-ray of the painful part of the arm or leg can be done.

3. Biopsy

In this procedure a small piece of tissue is taken from the bone to be examined under a microscope in the laboratory.

4. Bone scan

This is done to check if the cancer has spread to other bones.

5. CT (computerized tomography) scan of the chest

A CT scan uses x-rays to take pictures to see whether the cancer has spread to the chest.

6. MRI (magnetic resonance imaging) scan

A MRI scan uses magnetism to take pictures to see whether the cancer has spread to the surrounding muscles.

7. A PET (positron emission tomography) scan

A PET scan uses a mildly radioactive substance to measure the activity of cells in different parts of the body. It gives more information about the position of the tumor.

***

WHAT IS THE TREATMENT FOR OSTEOSARCOMA?

The treatment for Osteosarcoma includes:

1. Chemotherapy

Cytotoxic or anti-cancer drugs are given to destroy the cancer cells. These can be given before surgery to reduce the size of the tumor before the operation and also after surgery to reduce the chances of the tumor coming back.

2. Surgery

An operation is done while the patient is under general anesthesia. In early cases the surgeon can perform limb salvage surgery and spare the limb or in advanced cases the whole limb is amputated.

3. Radiotherapy

Radiotherapy can be given after the operation.

***

WHAT IS THE PROGNOSIS FOR OSTEOSARCOMA?

The prognosis for Osteosarcoma is better if the cancer has not spread to the lungs than if it has.

* * * * *

3

THROAT CANCER

WHAT IS THROAT CANCER?

Throat cancer is a term which covers tumors that develop in:

1. The throat or pharynx and are known as pharyngeal cancers

2. The larynx or voice box and are known as laryngeal cancers

3. The tonsils

***

WHAT CAUSES THROAT CANCER?

The cause of throat cancer is not known.

***

WHAT ARE THE RISK FACTORS FOR THROAT CANCER?

Risk factors for developing this malignancy include:

1. Smoking cigarettes

2. Chewing tobacco

3. Drinking too much alcohol

4. HPV or human papilloma virus which is thought to be transmitted by oral sex

5. Eating a diet without adequate fruits and vegetables

***

WHAT ARE THE SYMPTOMS OF THROAT CANCER?

Symptoms of throat cancer include:

1. Persistent sore throat

2. Persistent cough

3. Pain when swallowing (odynophagia) or difficulty swallowing (dysphagia)

4. Ear pain

5. Neck swelling

6. Voice changes like hoarseness

7. Weight loss

***

WHAT TESTS ARE DONE FOR THROAT CANCER?

Investigations for patients with throat cancer include:

1. Blood tests like a full blood count to check the blood level.

2. Laryngoscopy in which a doctor examines the throat with an instrument called a laryngoscope which has a lighted mirror.

2. Biopsy in which a small piece of tissue is taken to be examined under the microscope in the laboratory for the presence of cancer cells.

4. CT (computerized tomography) scan which uses x-rays to take pictures to see how far the cancer has spread.

5. MRI (magnetic resonance imaging) scan which uses magnetism to take pictures to see the extent of the tumor.

6. Barium swallow in which xrays of the esophagus are taken after a patient takes a drink that contains barium to line the organs.

***

WHAT IS THE TREATMENT FOR THROAT CANCER?

The treatment options for throat cancer depend on the location, size and stage of the tumor as well as the patient's age and general health. These treatment options include:

1. Surgery

An operation is done while the patient is under general anesthesia to remove the tumor. In the early stages only the tumor is removed. Laryngectomy or removal of the voice box is done if the tumor has spread into it. Pharyngectomy or removal of all or part of the throat is done if it has been affected by the tumor.

2. Radiotherapy or radiation therapy

High energy rays are used to destroy the cancer cells. In the very early and very advanced stages of throat cancer radiation therapy is usually the only therapy used. In the other stages it can either be combined with surgery or chemotherapy.

4. Chemotherapy

Cytotoxic or anti-cancer drugs are given to destroy the cancer cells. These are usually combined with radiation therapy or chemoradiation.

Patients receiving treatment for throat cancer have to stop smoking and drinking alcohol since they make the treatment less effective and increase the chances of the tumor recurring.

***

WHAT IS THE PROGNOSIS FOR THROAT CANCER?

The prognosis of throat cancer depends on the location, size and stage of the tumor as well as the patients age and general health.

***

HOW CAN THROAT CANCER BE PREVENTED?

Throat cancer can be prevented by the following measures:

1. Not smoking cigarettes

2. Not chewing tobacco

3. Taking minimal amounts of alcohol

4. Eating adequate amounts of fresh fruits and vegetables

* * * * *

4

CONGESTIVE HEART FAILURE

WHAT IS CONGESTIVE HEART FAILURE (CHF)?

Congestive heart failure is one of those cardiovascular or heart conditions in which the heart cannot pump enough oxygenated blood to meet the demands of the rest of the body.

***

WHAT CAUSES CONGESTIVE HEART FAILURE (CHF)?

Coronary artery disease, or narrowing of the heart's own blood vessels, is the most common cause congestive heart failure in the US since it causes around sixty percent of all cases.

The next most common cause is cardiomyopathy or heart muscle disease which can be caused by hypertension or high blood pressure, abusing alcohol or valvular heart disease.

Other causes of this chronic heart condition include congenital heart diseases, severe anemia and thyroid disorders.

***

WHAT ARE THE SYMPTOMS OF CONGESTIVE HEART FAILURE (CHF)?

Patients with CHF can develop symptoms of right heart or right ventricular failure, left heart or left ventricular failure and biventricular or right and left heart failure.

Symptoms of congestive heart failure that develop as a result of left ventricular failure include dyspnea or shortness of breath which occurs as a result of pulmonary vascular congestion with pooling of fluid in the lungs.

This difficulty in breathing can be exertional dyspnea which occurs when the patient is physically active or paroxysmal nocturnal dyspnea which occurs when the patient is lying in bed at night or in severe cases of heart failure, it can even occur at rest.

Right heart failure symptoms include ascites or collection of fluid in the abdomen as well as edema or swelling of the legs due to fluid retention. Other symptoms of congestive heart failure that arise as a result of right ventricular failure include anorexia or loss of appetite and fatigue.

Nocturia or passing urine many times during the night is another of the congestive heart failure symptoms which develops as a result of increased blood flow to the kidneys when the patient is lying down.

***

WHAT ARE THE SIGNS OF CONGESTIVE HEART FAILURE (CHF)?

On examination, signs of congestive heart failure include tachycardia or a rapid heart rate, tachypnea or an increased respiration rate, a third heart sound and pulmonary rales.

Distended neck veins as well as an enlarged, tender liver are other signs of congestive heart failure.

WHAT TESTS ARE DONE FOR CONGESTIVE HEART FAILURE (CHF)?

Investigations for patients with congestive heart failure include an echocardiogram which is done to diagnose the condition and to monitor ventricular function.

Other imaging investigations include chest x-rays which may reveal cardiomegaly or an enlarged heart as well as pulmonary congestion.

Laboratory tests done for patients with congestive heart failure include a complete blood count to check for anemia or a low blood count as well as kidney function and thyroid function tests.

***

WHAT IS THE TREATMENT FOR CONGESTIVE HEART FAILURE (CHF)?

Comprehensive congestive heart failure treatment comprises of treating any existing underlying cause such as anemia as well as symptomatic therapy.

Medications such as diuretics like furosemide which increase the excretion of water by the kidneys are part of the symptomatic congestive heart failure treatment.

Other medications used include angiotensin converting enzyme inhibitors such as captopril as well as digoxin which increases the heart's contractility and helps it pump better.

Surgical congestive heart failure treatment is reserved for severe cases which are unresponsive to medical management and thus require a heart transplant.

***

WHAT IS THE PROGNOSIS FOR CONGESTIVE HEART FAILURE (CHF)?

Being diagnosed with this commonly chronic heart condition does not signify impending death since a patient can improve their congestive heart failure prognosis by reducing their salt intake, exercising under supervision, loosing excess weight and taking their medications faithfully.

* * * * *

5

LEGIONNAIRE'S DISEASE

WHAT IS LEGIONNAIRE'S DISEASE

Legionnaire's disease, which is also called legionellosis, is a type of lung infection which can be fatal if it is not treated promptly.

This infection is called Legionnaire's disease because it was first identified after an outbreak occurred in 1976 in a hotel that was hosting an American legionnaires conference.

***

WHAT CAUSES LEGIONNAIRE'S DISEASE?

Legionnaire's disease is caused by a gram negative bacteria called Legionella pneumophila which lives in soil and freshwater streams, rivers, and lakes.

A person develops Legionnaire's disease when they inhale the bacteria in water droplets or mist from air conditioners, cooling towers, hot tubs, showers, faucets, whirlpools, swimming pools, nebulizers, physical therapy equipment and even mist sprayers in stores.

Legionnaire's disease can also be transmitted when water containing the bacteria enters the lungs. This can occur during choking while drinking.

Contaminated tap water has also been responsible for Legionnaire's disease in babies after water births.

Legionnaire's disease can also be contracted from working with soils with the bacteria.

Legionnaire's disease is not contagious since it cannot be spread from person to person like other types of chest infections like pulmonary tuberculosis (PTB).

Note that this bacteria also causes a minor flu-like illness called Pontiac fever which clears on its own without the use of antibiotics.

***

WHAT ARE THE RISK FACTORS FOR DEVELOPING LEGIONNAIRE'S DISEASE?

Persons who are more likely to develop Legionnaire's disease when exposed to the bacteria include:

1. Those who are 65 years old or older

2. Smokers

3. Persons with chronic lung diseases such as asthma and emphysema

4. Persons with cancers such as lung cancer

5. Persons with other serious diseases like diabetes, heart disease and kidney disease

6. Persons with a weak immune system due to HIV/AIDS or due to chemotherapy or due to taking medications to prevent organ rejection after transplants as well as taking corticosteroids such as prednisone

7. Persons working in cooling towers of air conditioning systems.

Most of the outbreaks of Legionnaire's disease have been linked to large buildings such as nursing homes, hotels and hospitals due to their complex air conditioning systems. Cruise ships whirlpools as well as decorative fountains have also been linked to outbreaks.

***

WHAT ARE THE SYMPTOMS OF LEGIONNAIRE'S DISEASE?

Symptoms of Legionnaire's disease usually develop from 2 days to 2 weeks after exposure to the bacteria. These symptoms include:

1. Initial symptoms like chills, a high fever which can pass 104 F (40 C), muscle pains and headaches.

2. These are then usually followed by cough which may be productive of blood stained sputum within 2 to 3 days. There may also be associated chest pain and shortness of breath.

3. Patients may also develop fatigue and anorexia or loss of appetite as well as nausea, vomiting and diarrhea. Some patients also develop confusion and difficulties concentrating.

In addition to infecting the lungs, the legionella bacteria also infect wounds which come in contact with the contaminated water.

***

WHAT INVESTIGATIONS ARE DONE FOR LEGIONNAIRE'S DISEASE?

Laboratory investigations done for patients with Legionnaire's disease include:

1. Urinary antigen test which checks for the presence of the Legionella pneumophila bacteria antigens in the urine and in the pleural fluid surrounding the lungs.

2. Direct fluorescent antibody DFA which tests for the presence of the bacteria in body fluid samples from the chest. A negative test does not rule out Legionnaire's disease.

3. Sputum tests which may reveal many polymorphonuclear leukocytes with sparse or absent organisms

4. Blood tests such as renal function tests which may reveal hyponatremia or low levels of sodium in the body.

Blood counts may also reveal leukocytosis (a high number of white blood cells). Erythrocyte sedimentation rates and C reactive protein levels are also usually elevated.

5. Lumbar puncture or spinal tap is done if symptoms such as confusion are present.

Radiological investigations done for patients with Legionnaire's disease include:

1. Chest xray is done as it can show the extent of the infection in the lungs.

2. CT scan of the brain is done in there are symptoms like confusion.

***

WHAT ARE THE DIFFERENTIAL DIAGNOSIS FOR LEGIONNAIRE'S DISEASE?

The differential diagnosis for Legionnaire's disease includes other chest infections like Mycoplasma pneumonias.

***

WHAT IS THE TREATMENT FOR LEGIONNAIRE'S DISEASE?

There treatment for Legionnaire's disease should be started early in order to prevent the development of complications.

This treatment includes:

1. Antibiotics such as Azithromycin (Zithromax) which is the drug of choice for children, Levofloxacin (Levaquin), Ciprofloxacin (Cipro), Doxycycline (Vibramycin), Trimethoprim and sulfamethoxazole (Bactrim)

Patients with collections of pus may need surgical drainage.

***

WHAT ARE THE COMPLICATIONS OF LEGIONNAIRE'S DISEASE?

Complications of Legionnaire's disease include:

1. Respiratory failure in which the lungs are incapable of providing the body with oxygenated blood.

Other respiratory complications include pulmonary cavities or holes in the lungs, empyema or collection of pus in the chest wall and emphysema.

2. Septic shock in which the blood pressure drops to such low levels that the flow of blood to the brain, kidneys and other vital organs is reduced.

3. Renal failure in which the kidneys are incapable of removing waste material from the blood.

4. Memory loss

5. Death

***

HOW CAN LEGIONNAIRE'S DISEASE BE PREVENTED?

Legionnaire's disease can be prevented by:

1. Maintaining water in water supply systems at the correct temperatures which should be either above 140 F (60 C) or below 68 F (20 C)

2. Using sterile water in nebulizers and physical therapy equipment

3. Disinfecting water systems like portable water distribution systems as well as pools and Jacuzzis.

4. Not smoking cigarettes

* * * * *

6

WEST NILE VIRUS

WHAT IS WEST NILE VIRUS?

West Nile Virus is a serious disease that causes seasonal epidemics in the summer that can continue spreading into fall.

***

WHAT CAUSES WEST NILE VIRUS?

West Nile Virus (WNV) is caused by a type of flavivirus which causes diseases in humans, birds, dogs and other animals.

This virus is spread to humans by the bite of infected Aedes, Anopheles and Culex mosquitoes. These mosquitoes get infected when they feed on infected birds.

Babies can also become infected with the WNV while in the uterus and after they are born while breastfeeding if their mothers are infected.

The West Nile Virus can also be spread by receiving blood transfusions and organ transplants from infected donors.

WNV is not spread through by shaking hands, touching and kissing an infected person.

***

WHAT ARE THE RISK FACTORS FOR DEVELOPING WEST NILE VIRUS?

Persons who are at a higher risk for developing West Nile Virus symptoms include:

1. Persons older than 50 years are more likely to develop the serious symptoms of WNV

2. Persons with a weakened immune system due to diseases such as HIV/AIDS or due to medications to prevent rejection of transplanted organs.

3. Persons who spend a lot of time working or playing outdoors especially at dawn and dusk.

***

WHAT ARE THE SYMPTOMS OF WEST NILE VIRUS?

Symptoms of West Nile Virus typically develop between 3 and 14 days after being bitten by the infected mosquito and include the following:

1. Neuroinvasive Disease

Less than 1 out of every 100 people infected with the WNV develop the serious neuroinvasive disease which means it affects the nervous system.

Symptoms of this neuroinvasive disease include a high fever, severe headaches, encephalitis (inflammation of the brain), meningitis (inflammation of the membranes surrounding the brain and spinal cord), West Nile poliomyelitis (inflammation of the spinal cord), neck stiffness, muscle weakness and paralysis, numbness, tremors, confusion, convulsions and coma.

These symptoms of the severe illness can last for weeks to months and even cause permanent neurological deficits.

2. Non-Neuroinvasive Disease

Around 1 out of every 5 people who are infected with WNV develop West Nile Fever or the non-neuroinvasive disease whose symptoms include fever, headaches, body pains, vomiting and fatigue. A few of these patients may also develop enlarged lymph glands, pain in their eyes and a rash on the back, chest and stomach. These symptoms of the mild illness can last for days to weeks.

3. Asymptomatic Infection

Around 4 out of every 5 people who are infected with the WNV do not develop any symptoms.

***

WHAT INVESTIGATIONS ARE DONE FOR WEST NILE VIRUS?

Laboratory investigations done for patients with West Nile Virus include:

1. Complete blood count which may have normal or high numbers of white blood cells.

2. Kidney function test may reveal hyponatremia or low sodium levels especially in patients who have developed encephalitis.

3. Cerebrospinal fluid (CSF) obtained by a spinal tap or lumbar puncture usually reveals increased protein and white blood cells with normal glucose levels.

4. MAC-ELISA or IgM antibody-capture enzyme linked immunosorbent assay can be used to detect antibodies to the WNV in the blood or CSF.

Radiological investigations done for patients with West Nile Virus include:

1. Magnetic Resonance Imaging (MRI) scans which may show enhancement of the membranes covering the brain in some patients infected with WNV.

WHAT ARE THE DIFFERENTIAL DIAGNOSIS FOR WEST NILE VIRUS?

The differential diagnosis for West Nile Virus include:

1. Poliomyelitis

2. Gullain-Barre Syndrome

***

WHAT IS THE TREATMENT FOR WEST NILE VIRUS?

Since there is no specific treatment for West Nile Virus, management of infected persons includes:

1. Supportive treatment for example in the form of intravenous fluids.

2. Rehabilitation programs for those who suffer brain damage from WNV encephalitis and meningitis. These can include physical therapists (to help with muscle weakness), speech therapists (to help them with speaking and swallowing), occupational therapists (to help them with dressing and feeding) and other professionals depending on the specific injury the patient has suffered.

***

WHAT ARE THE COMPLICATIONS OF WEST NILE VIRUS?

Complications of West Nile Virus include:

1. Permanent muscle weakness in some of those who develop the neuroinvasive disease.

2. Deep venous thrombosis or blood clotting in the leg veins. This can become fatal if the clot moves to the lungs as a pulmonary embolus.

3. Pressure ulcers or bed sores can develop in those who are bed ridden.

4. Death in those who develop the neuroinvasive disease.

HOW IS WEST NILE VIRUS PREVENTED?

West Nile Virus can be prevented by:

1. Avoiding mosquito bites by instituting personal protection measures. These include:

a. Applying insect repellents to exposed skin whenever one is going outdoors. These insect repellents should contain ingredients registered by the EPA as being effective such as DEET, Picaridin, Oil of Lemon Eucalyptus or PMD and IR3535.

b. Wearing long sleeved tops and long pants when going outdoors at dusk and at dawn because the mosquitoes are most active during those periods. When wearing thin garments consider spraying insect repellents on the garments since the mosquitoes can bite through the thin materials.

c. Keeping mosquitoes out of your house by having good screens on your doors and windows.

2. Preventing mosquito bites by establishing community based programs to control the mosquito population. These include:

a. Eradicating all potential mosquito breeding sites or where they can potentially lay their eggs by draining all containers with standing water such as open barrels, flower pots and wading pools.

b. Changing the water in pet dishes regularly to discard mosquito eggs before they hatch.

* * * * *

7

CRYPTOSPORIDIOSIS

WHAT IS CRYPTOSPORIDIOSIS?

Cryptosporidiosis is a disease caused by the protozoa Cryptosporidium parvum.

***

WHAT IS THE LIFE CYCLE OF THE CRYPTOSPORIDIOSIS PARASITE?

Humans are infested with these intestinal parasites by eating food and water contaminated with their oocysts or eggs.

Once ingested, the oocyts release sporozoites which change into trophozoites that replicate and produce more oocysts in the small intestines.

These oocyts are then excreted in the feces and the cycle continues.

***

WHO IS AT RISK FOR DEVELOPING CRYPTOSPORIDIOSIS?

Though cryptosporidiosis commonly affects immunocompromised persons or those with a weak immune system such as AIDS patients and transplant recipients, it seldom affects persons with a competent immune system.

Immunocompetent persons at risk of developing cryptosporidiosis include children aged less than five years in daycare facilities, their caregivers and other workers who might be exposed to feces, men who have sex with men as well as calf and other animal handlers.

***

WHAT ARE THE SYMPTOMS OF CRYPTOSPORIDIOSIS?

The incubation period of cryptosporidiosis is one week.

Symptoms of infection with these parasites in humans include watery diarrhea, abdominal pain and less frequently fever and nausea.

***

HOW IS THE DIAGNOSIS OF CRYPTOSPORIDIOSIS MADE?

Diagnosis of cryptosporidiosis is made by examining an acid fast stained stool sample for the Cryptosporidium parvum oocyts.

Antibody tests are also done to look for the parasites in human stool. An intestinal biopsy can also be done as a last resort.

***

WHAT IS THE TREATMENT FOR CRYPTOSPORIDIOSIS?

Immunocompetent patients with cryptosporidiosis only need supportive treatment such as fluids to prevent dehydration as the infestation is usually self limiting and resolves within two weeks.

The situation is very different for immunocompromised persons with cryptosporidiosis since they may continue having chronic diarrhea despite taking prescription medications such as paromomycin, spiramycin, nitazoxide and azithromycin which are used for its treatment because there is no effective cryptosporidiosis treatment. Patients with AIDS may benefit by taking combination antiretroviral therapy.

***

WHAT ARE THE COMPLICATIONS OF CRYPTOSPORIDIOSIS?

Complications of infestation with these intestinal parasites include cholecystitis of inflammation of the gall bladder, malabsorption or inadequate absorption of nutrients from the intestines as well as wasting.

***

HOW CAN CRYPTOSPORIDIOSIS BE PREVENTED?

Prevention of cryptosporidiosis is therefore better than waiting to seek a cure especially for immunocompromised persons because of its complications and the fact that no effective cryptosporidiosis treatment exists. This can be done by instituting proper hygiene and sanitation policies such as hand washing as well as using water filters with pore sizes of less than one micrometer such as those certified to NSF/ANSI Standard 53 or 55 or 58.

Boiling drinking water for more than sixty seconds is also useful since these human parasites are resistant to the chlorine concentrations used for water treatment.

* * * * *

8

CYCLOSPORA

WHAT CAUSES CYCLOSPORA?

Cyclospora or cyclosporiasis is caused by a protozoa called Cyclospora cayetanensis.

This parasite, which has just once cell, usually infests humans when they swallow its oocyst or inactive form. The swallowed oocyst becomes active and causes the symptoms associated with cyclospora. After several cycles of asexual reproduction, they reproduce sexually and produce oocysts which are excreted in the stool.

If the hygiene levels of the infested person and their surroundings are low, the stool with the oocysts contaminates human food and water sources and the cycle continues as more people ingest the oocysts.

***

WHAT ARE THE RISK FACTORS FOR CYCLOSPORA?

The main risk factor for developing cyclospora is eating food or drinking water that has been contaminated with feces with the oocysts.

Many cases have been reported to have developed after eating imported fresh fruits and vegetables like raspberries, lettuce, snow peas and even herbs like basil.

***

WHAT ARE THE SYMPTOMS OF CYCLOSPORA?

Symptoms of cyclospora include:

1. Watery diarrhea which can be explosive and lead to dehydration

2. Nausea and vomiting

3. Low grade fever

4. Loss of appetite

5. Fatigue

6. Muscle aches

7. Weight loss

8. Bloating, flatulence and burping

These symptoms can develop anywhere from 2 days to 2 weeks after eating the contaminated food.

Symptoms of cyclospora in patients with compromised immune systems can be more severe and can even include upper abdominal pain on the right side.

***

WHAT TESTS ARE DONE FOR CYCLOSPORA?

Investigations for patients with cyclospora include:

1. Stool tests to check for the presence of oocytes. The stool may have to be concentrated since the parasites are not present in large numbers.

2. Polymerase chain reaction (PCR) test can also be done to check for cyclospora DNA in stool.

WHAT IS THE TREATMENT FOR CYCLOSPORA?

In healthy persons, the disease is usually self limiting and resolves in 2-7 days. Treatment for such cases of cyclospora is usually supportive and includes:

1. Fluids which can be taken orally (by mouth) or even given intravenously (in the veins).

2. Medications for the vomiting

Persons who develop severe cases or prolonged symptoms are treated with the antibiotic trimethoprim-sulfamethoxazole (Bactrim or Septra) for 7 to 10 days.

Ciprofloxacin (Cipro) or nitazoxanide (Alinia) are used for those who have sulfa allergy.

***

HOW CAN CYCLOSPORA BE PREVENTED?

Cyclospora can be prevented by thoroughly washing all fresh produce before eating it. The fruits and vegetables should then be dried with a paper towel since the cyclospora can be quite difficult to dislodge from the produce.

* * * * *

9

POLYMYALGIA RHEUMATICA

WHAT CAUSES POLYMYALGIA RHEUMATICA?

Polymyalgia Rheumatica is an inflammatory disease which usually affects people above the age of 50 years. It affects more women than men. The cause of polymyalgia rheumatic is unknown.

***

WHAT ARE THE SYMPTOMS OF POLYMYALGIA RHEUMATICA?

Symptoms and signs of Polymyalgia Rheumatica include:

1. Pain of the neck, pectoral girdle (shoulder and upper arm muscles)and pelvic girdle (hip and thigh muscles) which can be severe.

2. Stiffness of these muscle groups which is associated with morning stiffness and stiffness after periods of inactivity.

3. The examination of the musculoskeletal system is normal though the muscle power may appear slightly reduced if the patient is examined while in pain.

4. Constitutional symptoms such a weight loss due to loss of appetite, fever and general malaise may also be present.

5. Around 15% of patients with polymyalgia rheumatica also have temporal (giant cell) arteritis. Symptoms of temporal arteritis include headaches, scalp tenderness, and visual disturbances which may lead to blindness.

***

WHAT INVESTIGATIONS ARE DONE FOR POLYMYALGIA RHEUMATICA?

There is no diagnostic test for polymyalgia rheumatic though laboratory investigations that can be done for patients suspected to have Polymyalgia Rheumatica include:

1. Hemogram may reveal a normochromic-normocytic anemia.

2. Erythrocyte sedimentation rate (ESR) which is usually elevated.

3. A temporal artery biopsy should be done on patients suspected of having temporal arteritis.

***

WHAT IS THE TREATMENT FOR POLYMYALGIA RHEUMATICA?

There treatment for Polymyalgia Rheumatica includes corticosteroids.

Patients with temporal arteritis should be started on high doses of prednisone since it can lead to blindness. Patients with uncomplicated polymyalgia rheumatica can be managed with lower doses of prednisone.

* * * * *

10

SARCOIDOSIS

WHAT IS SARCOIDOSIS?

Sarcoidosis is a disease which affects many organs in the body like the lungs, lymph glands, eyes, kidneys and the skin.

It is characterized by granulomas or collections of inflammatory cells in these organs.

***

WHAT CAUSES SARCOIDOSIS?

The exact cause of sarcoidosis is not known.

It is however known that it develops as a result of the body having an abnormal immune response to something that is also not yet known.

Substances suspected to trigger this abnormal response include inhaled bacteria, viruses, dust and chemicals.

***

WHO GETS SARCOIDOSIS?

Risk factors for developing sarcoidosis include:

1.Persons aged between 20 and 40 years of age

2. Being a woman since it affects more women than men

3. Being African Americans since it affects more African Americans than Caucasians. It is also more severe and more likely to cause lung complications in African Americans.

4. Having a family history of sarcoidosis since some families appear to have a genetic predisposition to developing sarcoidosis.

***

WHAT ARE THE SYMPTOMS OF SARCOIDOSIS?

Symptoms of sarcoidosis depend on the organ affected. For example patients with:

1. Lung involvement can develop cough, wheezing, chest pain and shortness of breath.

2. Lymph gland involvement can develop painful and swollen glands in the neck, armpits, groin and inside the chest.

3. Bone involvement can develop pain in the hands or feet due to cysts in the bones.

4. Heart involvement can develop palpitations or abnormal heart beats and heart failure.

5. Skin involvement can develop a reddish rash on the shins which may be associated with painful swellings or they can develop ulcers on the nose, cheeks and ears or hyperpigmentation (the skin getting darker) or hypopigmentation (the skin getting lighter).

6. Eye involvement can develop red eyes, teary eyes, blurred vision, light sensitivity and pain in the eyes.

Other symptoms of sarcoidosis include fatigue, fever, weight loss, swollen and painful joints, kidney stone formation, hearing loss, convulsions, depression, dementia and psychosis.

Sarcoidosis is one of those diseases in which patients can present very differently. For example some patients rapidly develop very severe symptoms while others do not develop any symptoms despite multiple organs being affected. In fact, a good number of patients discover that they have sarcoidosis when they have a chest x-ray done for a totally unrelated reason.

***

WHAT TESTS ARE DONE FOR SARCOIDOSIS?

Investigations for patients with sarcoidosis include:

1. Chest x-rays which may reveal swollen nodes in the chest (lymphadenopathy) or cloudiness in the lung fields (pulmonary infiltrates).

2. CT scans of the chest which give more information on the extent of the disease in the chest.

3. Pulmonary function tests (breathing tests) since these evaluate how well the lungs are working.

4. Bronchoscopy with biopsy which involves passing a small tube with a tiny camera into the lungs to inspect them and take a sample of the tissue for further testing.

5. Kidney function tests to evaluate how well the lungs are working.

6. Skin biopsies to confirm the diagnosis.

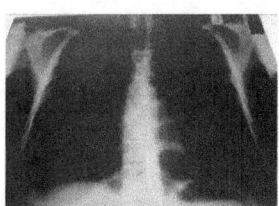

***

WHAT IS THE TREATMENT FOR SARCOIDOSIS?

There is no definitive treatment for sarcoidosis but this is not bad news for all patients since it can resolve spontaneously.

In addition to the disease getting better without treatment, many persons have mild symptoms which do not need treatment.

The treatment that is given for those patients who need it is mainly what is known as symptomatic treatment. This is treatment that only reduces the symptoms since there is no cure for sarcoidosis.

Symptomatic treatment for sarcoidosis involves the use of:

1. Oxygen therapy

2. Corticosteroids like prednisone to reduce inflammation in the affected organs. These are especially beneficial in reducing symptoms of cough and fatigue.

3. Nonsteroidal anti-inflammatory drugs (NSAIDS) like ibuprofen are used by patients with joint pains and fever.

4. Medications like methotrexate, azathioprine, plaquenil and infliximab.

5. Rehabilitation

6. Organ transplants when the kidney or lungs fail.

In addition to the above treatment, patients with sarcoidosis should ensure that they:

1. Eat a balanced diet with plenty of fresh fruits and vegetables.

8. Drink 10 glasses of pure water each day.

4. Sleep for at least 6 hours each night

5. Exercise regularly

6. Maintain a healthy body weight

7. Stop smoking

Patients with high levels of calcium in their blood or urine should avoid foods that are rich in calcium like milk, cheese and other dairy products.

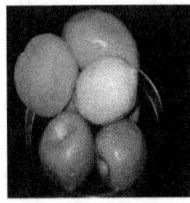 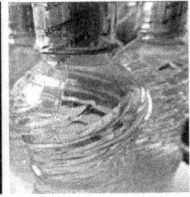 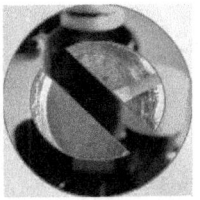

***

WHAT IS THE PROGNOSIS FOR SARCOIDOSIS?

Being diagnosed with sarcoidosis does not signify impending death since in many patients the disease resolves on its own.

A minority, around 20-30%, develop permanent lung damage which may result in difficulty breathing.

Other complications of sarcoidosis include blindness and kidney failure.

Very few patients die because of sarcoidosis and those who do usually have complications in their heart like abnormal heart rhythms or in their lungs and brain.

* * * * *

11

ALCOHOLIC LIVER CIRRHOSIS

WHAT IS ALCOHOLIC LIVER CIRRHOSIS?

Alcoholic liver cirrhosis which is also known as Laennec's cirrhosis, is a relatively common alcoholic liver disease.

***

WHAT CAUSES ALCOHOLIC LIVER CIRRHOSIS?

Alcoholic cirrhosis of the liver is caused by abusing alcohol usually daily and for over 10 years.

***

WHAT ARE THE SYMPTOMS OF ALCOHOLIC LIVER CIRRHOSIS?

Patients with alcoholic liver cirrhosis initially may have no symptoms (asymptomatic).

But, as the disease progresses, alcoholic liver disease symptoms develop and include abdominal discomfort or pain and abdominal distension as a substantial amount of fluid collects in the abdomen (ascites).

Other liver cirrhosis symptoms include loss of appetite (anorexia), fatigue and jaundice (yellow eyes). Patients with massive ascites may also complain of dyspnea (difficulty breathing).

***

WHAT ARE THE SIGNS OF ALCOHOLIC LIVER CIRRHOSIS?

On examination, patients with alcoholic cirrhosis of the liver may have signs of liver damage such as jaundice (yellowness of eyes), spider veins, gynecomastia breast enlargement in men) and testicular atrophy (shrunken testicles).

***

WHAT TESTS ARE DONE FOR ALCOHOLIC LIVER CIRRHOSIS?

Tests done on patients with alcoholic liver damage include liver function tests and a liver biopsy.

A diagnostic paracentesis is done by removing a small amount of fluid from the abdominal cavity to determine the cause of the ascites.

Ascitic fluid resulting from liver cirrhosis is usually clear, straw-colored and a transudate. This means it has a protein concentration of less than 3 g/dl and a white blood cell count of less than 300/ul.

Abdominal ultrasounds or CT scans also are done for imaging purposes and also because they can detect much smaller quantities of fluid than those detected on physical examination in patients with alcohol liver disease.

***

WHAT IS THE TREATMENT FOR ALCOHOLIC LIVER CIRRHOSIS?

Treatment for patients with this alcoholic liver disease should start with stopping taking alcohol since continued intake worsens the prognosis.

Dietary sodium restriction to 40mEq/day as well as bed rest are also important. The later in some cases helps reduce aldosterone production in the body.

Diuretics are also used in liver cirrhosis treatment. The diuretic of choice is spironolactone which is a potassium sparing diuretic. Loop diuretics such as furosemide and thiazide diuretics such us hydrochlorothiazide can also be added to the treatment of alcoholic liver cirrhosis.

Therapeutic paracentesis or putting a needle into the abdominal cavity and drawing out the fluid can also be done if the ascitics is massive and is causing respiratory embarrassment. If this is done, the patient should receive intravenous albumin concomitantly to prevent intravascular volume depletion.

Surgical management of alcoholic cirrhosis of the liver includes the use of transjugular intrahepatic portosystemic shunts (TIPS) which connect the portal and hepatic veins to decrease portal hypertension and ascites. Other surgical shunts such as the LeVeen and Denver shunts are also used in resistant cases. Liver transplants can also be considered.

* * * * *

12

DRY DROWNING

WHAT IS DRY DROWNING?

The term dry drowning is used to refer to a situation in which a person drowns when they are not submerged in water.

This is due to the fact that dry drowning can occur anywhere from 1 hour to 1 day after the person finishes swimming or bathing.

***

WHAT CAUSES DRY DROWNING?

Dry drowning in caused by water entering the lungs when a person inhales or swallows it.

The water in the lungs causes the airways to develop spasms, constrict and close up. This results in reduced oxygen supply to the brain and other organs and subsequently death if not attended to promptly.

A person does not need to inhale large amounts of water to dry drown since it can occur when children are playing in bathtubs, hot tubs, spas and buckets of water.

WHAT ARE THE RISK FACTORS?

Factors that increase a person's chances of dry drowning include:

1. Swimming for the first time

2. Being a poor swimmer

3. Being injured while swimming

4. Suffering from lung problems like asthma

5. Drinking alcohol or taking sedatives before swimming

6. Not using life jackets

***

WHAT ARE THE SYMPTOMS OF DRY DROWNING?

Symptoms of dry drowning develop as a result of reduced oxygen supply to the brain and include:

1. Difficulty breathing or shortness of breath

2. Excessive fatigue

3. Changes in behavior like confusion, having accidents in the pool, being abnormally combative or moody

4. Losing consciousness

5. Persistent cough, chest pain

6. Cold clammy skin

7. Changes in skin color with the skin becoming pale or bluish or grayish

***

WHAT IS THE TREATMENT FOR DRY DROWNING?

The treatment for dry drowning includes:

1. Endotracheal intubation in which the doctor passes a tube into the patient's lungs to supply them with oxygen.

***

HOW CAN DRY DROWNING BE PREVENTED?

Dry drowning can be prevented by the following measures:

1. Watching children keenly when swimming or bathing to ensure that they do not inhale water.

2. Taking children to be examined by a doctor if they have near drowning experiences when swimming or bathing even if they seem normal since dry drowning can occur up to24 hours after the incident.

3. Teaching children how to swim and instructing them to always swim with a friend.

4. Parents and guardians of children learning CPR (cardio-pulmonary resuscitation).

* * * * *

13

PROSOPAGNOSIA

WHAT IS PROSOPAGNOSIA?

Prosopagnosia is a condition in which a person cannot recognize faces.

Prosopagnosia, which comes from the Greek words for face "prosopon" and lack of knowledge "agnosia" is also known as facial agnosia or face blindness.

This face blindness varies from severe cases who are not able to recognize their own face or even differentiate a human face from an inanimate object to mild cases who are unable to recognize faces of acquaintances but can teach themselves to memorize faces.

In some cases, prosopagnosia is also associated with inability to recognize animals, cars and places.

Some prosopagnosics are also unable to recognize other facial aspects like a person's age, gender and even their emotions.

***

WHAT CAUSES PROSOPAGNOSIA?

Prosopagnosia is associated with damage or dysfunction of a part of the brain known as the right fusiform gyrus. This is the part that synchronizes facial perception and memory.

For purposes of describing its causes, prosopagnosia can be divided into developmental and acquired prosopagnosia.

Developmental prosopagnosia occurs before a person develops adult face recognition abilities. These abilities usually mature by the teenage years. Acquired prosopagnosia occurs after a person has developed adult face recognition abilities.

Causes of Developmental Prosopagnosia include:

1. Genetic causes and these cases run in families

2. Brain damage prenatally (before birth) or during birth or in childhood

3. Severe eye problems in childhood

Causes of Acquired Prosopagnosia include:

1. Brain damage from head injury, strokes and degenerative diseases

***

WHAT ARE THE SYMPTOMS OF PROSOPAGNOSIA?

Symptoms of Prosopagnosia include:

1. Relying on the voice, hair, body shape, clothing, jewelry, gait and other characteristics to recognize a person

2. Difficulty following movies, plays and TV programs because of inability to recognize the characters

3. Avoidance of social situations due to the problems associated with being labeled rude because of the inability to recognize and

acknowledge friends and acquaintances. Some prosopagnosics have even developed social anxiety disorder.

***

WHAT TESTS ARE DONE FOR PROSOPAGNOSIA?

Research centers usually offer Face Recognition Tests to identify prosopagnosics.

***

WHAT IS THE TREATMENT FOR PROSOPAGNOSIA?

The treatment for prosopagnosia involves developing compensatory techniques for recognizing faces. These compensatory strategies can include using a person's striking physical characteristics or their physical location. Examples of the latter include identifying a person by their work cubicle or their sitting location in a lecture hall.

***

WHAT IS THE PROGNOSIS FOR PROSOPAGNOSIA?

The prognosis depends on the severity of the prosopagnosia and how well a person develops compensatory mechanisms. Mild prosopagnosics who learn to memorize faces therefore have a better prognosis than those with severe prosopagnosia and cannot differentiate a face fron an object.

* * * * *

ABOUT THE AUTHOR

Dr. Miriam Kinai is a medical doctor.

You can visit her blog at http://www.MyBlogBookClub.com or follow her on twitter at http://twitter.com/AlmasiHealth

Email enquiries to almasihealthcare@yahoo.com with BOOKS as your subject.

HERBS AND SPICES FOR THE COOK, HEALER AND BEAUTICIAN

Herbs and Spices for the Cook, Healer and Beautician uses color pictures and clear explanations to teach you about more than 70 healing herbs and spices.

You will learn about their:

* Therapeutic (healing) uses

* Drug interactions

* Contraindications (when not to use them)

* Cooking tips

* Beauty tips

*****

INTERNATIONAL GOURMET HERB AND SPICE BLENDS

International Gourmet Herb and Spice Blends teaches you how to prepare exotic herb and spice blends from around the world. You will discover the recipes for:

* Barbecue Rub, Cajun, Apple Pie and Pumpkin Pie Spice Mixes from America

* Pudding Spice Mix from Britain

* 5 Spice Mix from China

* Berbere Spice Mix from Ethiopia

* Curry Powder and Garam Masala from India

* Bouquet Garni, Herbs de Provence and Quatre Epices from France

* Herb Mix from Italy

* Jerk Seasoning from Jamaica

* Shichimi Togarashi from Japan

* Pilau Spice Blend from Kenya

* Chili Powder from Mexico

* Baharat Spice Blend from the Middle East

* Ras El Hanout from Morocco

*****

THE QUICK GOURMET CHEF

The Quick Gourmet is an essential culinary skills cookbook which teaches how to make simple, divine dishes.

You will learn how to make:

* Hot Chocolate Mixes and Drinks

* Hot Chai Tea Mixes and Drinks

* Hot Coffee Mixes and Drinks

* Sensational Smoothies

* Non-Dairy Smoothies

* Chocolate Covered Strawberries

* Chocolate Truffles

* Healthy Chicken Salads

* Healthy Tuna Salads

* Savory Salsas

* Herb Butter

* Cheese Dips and Sauces

* Gourmet Sandwiches

* Perfect Hard Boiled Eggs

* A Cheese Board

* Natural Food Color

*****

HOW TO STYLE AND PHOTOGRAPH FOOD

Regardless of whether you are an aspiring food blogger or you want to make money online selling stock photos, How To Style and Photograph Food, uses color pictures and clear explanations to teach you the food photography tips that can help you improve your digital camera photography skills so that you can begin photographing food like a pro.

You will learn:

* The equipment that you need

* How to set up the lighting

* How to prepare the stage

* How to style the food

* How to shoot the food

*****

HOW TO MAKE NATURAL SKIN CARE PRODUCTS VOLUME 1

How To Make Natural Skin Care Products Volume 1 by Dr Miriam Kinai is filled with recipes for making organic bath and body products for normal, sensitive, oily and dry skin types as well as therapeutic products to manage mature skin, prematurely aging skin, cellulite, eczema, psoriasis, ringworms, dandruff, thinning hair, menopausal symptoms, pre-menstrual tension (PMS), painful periods, arthritis, stress, sadness or depression, mental exhaustion and insomnia.

This book also teaches you the best vegetable oils, essential oils, natural butters and herbs to use when making products for different skin types physical conditions. You will learn how to make:

* Bath bombs

* Bath melts

* Bath salts

* Bath teas

* Body butters

* Body lotions

* Body scrubs

* Healing balms and body creams

* Herb infused oils

* Natural soap

How to Make Natural Skin Care Products Volume 1 will leave you with a clear understanding of how to make bath and beauty products to use in your home or to give as gifts or to sell and make money.

*****

ORGANIC SKIN CARE PRODUCT INGREDIENTS

Organic Skin Care Product Ingredients teaches you about the different natural substances that can be used to create natural bath and beauty products to use in your home or to give as gifts to your loved ones or to sell and make money.

You will learn about:

* Natural butters

* Natural clays

* Natural colorants

* Natural exfoliants

* Natural fragrances

* Natural oils

* Natural preservatives

*****

THE ESSENTIALS OF AROMATHERAPY ESSENTIAL OILS

The Essentials of Aromatherapy Essential Oils by Dr Miriam Kinai teaches you how to use aromatherapy oils to improve your physical, mental and emotional well being.

The author's experience as a medical doctor and clinical aromatherapy practitioner have enabled her to write a highly informative guide for those who want to utilize the healing benefits of these natural plant essences.

You will discover:

* The safety information and therapeutic uses of 18 essential oils

* How to blend essential oils

* The characteristics and uses of 14 carrier oils

* How to Dilute Essential Oils with Carrier Oils

* How to Use Essential Oils

* Cautionary Measures when using Essential Oils

* Numerous Essential Oil Recipes for bath products as well as skin care and hair care products

The Essentials of Aromatherapy Essential Oils will leave you with a clear understanding of how you can safely use aromatherapy essential oils to heal yourself naturally.

*****

CARRIER OILS GUIDE

Carrier Oils Guide teaches you the characteristics, health benefits and uses of commonly used carrier oils. You will learn about:

* Apricot Kernel Oil

* Avocado Oil

* Borage Seed Oil

* Calendula Oil

* Carrot Seed Oil

* Castor Oil

* Evening Primrose Oil

* Fractionated Coconut Oil

* Jojoba

* Olive Oil

* Rosehip Oil

* Sunflower Oil

* Sweet Almond Oil

* Virgin Coconut Oil

* Useful formulas for Diluting Essential Oils with Carrier Oils

*****

MEDICAL AROMATHERAPY FOR HEALTH PROFESSIONALS

Medical Aromatherapy for Healthcare Professionals by Dr Miriam Kinai teaches you how to use essential oils to treat physical diseases and emotional disorders.

The author's experience as a medical doctor and clinical aromatherapy practitioner have enabled her to write a highly informative guide for those who want to utilize the healing benefits of these natural plant essences.

You will discover how to use essential oils to:

* Treat skin diseases like acne, eczema and psoriasis

* Treat other physical diseases like high blood pressure, arthritis, coughs and colds

* Manage mental and emotional conditions like anxiety, depression, anger and stress

* Relieve the symptoms of menopause and premenstrual tension

* Lessen insomnia and impotence

Medical Aromatherapy for Healthcare Professionals is therefore an essential resource for holistic healthcare practitioners like massage therapists, naturopaths and herbalists.

It is also a useful resource for conventional medicine healthcare providers like physicians and nurses who want to begin practicing integrative medicine and for patients who want to improve their health naturally by using aromatherapy oils.

*****

AROMATHERAPY COURSE

Aromatherapy Course by Dr Miriam Kinai tutors you on how to use essential oils to improve your physical, mental and emotional well being.

The author's experience as a medical doctor and clinical aromatherapy practitioner have enabled her to create a highly informative course on how to use these natural plant essences.

You will learn:

* The safety information and therapeutic uses of essential oils like clary sage, eucalyptus, geranium, grapefruit, lavender, lemon, lemongrass, marjoram, orange (sweet), patchouli, peppermint, Roman chamomile, rose, rosemary, sandalwood, spearmint, tea tree and ylang ylang.

* The safety information and therapeutic uses of carrier oils like apricot kernel oil, avocado oil, borage seed oil, calendula oil, carrot seed oil, castor oil, evening primrose oil, fractionated coconut oil, jojoba, olive oil, rosehip oil, sunflower oil, sweet almond oil and virgin coconut oil.

* How to blend essential oils

* How to dilute essential oils with carrier oils

* How to administer essential oils

* How to make natural healing products from numerous aromatherapy recipes

* How to utilize the healing benefits of essentials oils even if you do not have prior training in aromatherapy

The Aromatherapy Course will leave you with a clear understanding of how you can heal yourself and your family naturally by using essentials oils on your body and in your home.

*****

DEALING WITH DEPRESSION NATURALLY

Dealing with Depression Naturally presents a holistic approach to managing depression with natural antidepressants. You will learn how to treat depression with:

* Aromatherapy

* Art therapy

* Christian Biblical principles

* Chromotherapy

* Diet therapy

* Eco-therapy

* Herbal therapy

* Home decor therapy

* Music therapy

* Phototherapy

* Exercise therapy

* Self-Psychotherapy

* Social therapy

* Talk therapy

* Vitamin therapy

* Writing therapy

*****

CHRISTIAN LIFE COACHING HANDBOOK

Christian Life Coaching Handbook offers a Biblical approach to managing different aspects of life.

You will learn:

* Christian anger management

* Christian conflict resolution

* Christian depression treatment

* Christian goal setting

* Christian marital stress management

* Christian stress management

* How to assert yourself

* How to defeat fear

* How to love yourself

* How to overcome shyness

* How to resist temptation

* How to stop being a people pleaser

*****

CHRISTIAN PERSONAL FINANCE

Christian Personal Finance teaches Biblical principles of money management.

You will learn:

* Christian financial stress management from people who were dealing with money stress like the Acts 3 beggar or credit issues like the widow in second Kings.

* Biblical prosperity principles from wealthy men and women of God like Isaac and the Proverbs 31 woman.

* Bible verses to use as spiritual warfare prayers and as Christian finance affirmations and Christian money meditations.

*****

ANTHOLOGY OF CHRISTIAN BIBLE SERMONS

Anthology of Christian Bible Sermons is a compilation of more than 20 Biblical rhema teachings which include:

* A New Christmas Message

* A New Easter Message

* Are You A Flamboyant Fig Tree Christian?

* Biblical Lessons for Purim from Queen Esther

* Can God Help Me If I Am Surrounded By Enemies?

* How Badly Do You Really Want It?

* Seed Words And The Powerful Tongue

* Spiritual AIDS

* The Three Levels Of Getting Lost

* Why Does God Allow Suffering?

* Your Life Is Your Ministry And Your Storm Is Your Message

* A Perfect God, Imperfect People, and Perfect Plans

* We Are Not Ignorant of His Devices

* How to Prepare for a Dangerous Journey

* Yes, God Can

* How to Serve the Body of Christ

* Conduits of God

* Go Back? Stand Still? Move Forward? Drown?

*****

CHRISTIAN SPIRITUAL WARFARE

Christian Spiritual Warfare teaches you the awesome Bible verses you can use as spiritual warfare prayers, Christian affirmations and in your Christian meditation sessions as you fight your spiritual battles.

You will learn how to fight for the following with Bible verses:

* Marriage * Children * Health

* Christian Faith * Christian Ministry

* Country

* Finances * Job * Business

* Peace of Mind * Restoration * Self Esteem * Self Love

You will also learn how to fight against the following with Bible verses:

* Addiction * Temptation

* Being Single * Infertility

* Opposition * Oppression

* Worry * Fear

* Feelings of Condemnation * Confusion

* Danger * Death * Despair * Discouragement

* Impatience * Insomnia * Laziness * Loneliness

* Poverty * Pride * Sadness

* Vengeance * Weakness

* A Foul Mouth * Lying

*****

DARK SKIN DERMATOLOGY COLOR ATLAS

Dark Skin Dermatology Color Atlas is filled with clear explanations and color photos of skin, hair, and nail diseases affecting people with skin of color or Fitzpatrick skin types IV, V, and VI.

Topics covered include Acne Vulgaris, Alopecia Areata, Anal Warts, Angioedema, Aphthous Ulcers, Atopic Dermatitis, Blastomycosis, Blister Beetle Dermatitis or Nairobi Fly Dermatitis, Cellulitis, Chronic Ulcers, Confetti Hypopigmentation, Cutaneous T Cell Lymphoma, Cutaneous Tuberculosis, Dermatitis Artefacta, Erythema Nodosum,

Exfoliative Erythroderma, Gianotti Crosti Syndrome, Hand Dermatitis, Hemangioma, Herpes Zoster, Ichthyosis, Ingrown Toenails, Irritant Contact Dermatitis, Kaposi Sarcoma, Keloids, Keratoderma Blenorrhagica, Klippel Trenaunay Weber Syndrome, Leishmaniasis, Leprosy, Leukonychia, Lichen Nitidus, Lichen Planus,

Lichenoid Drug Eruption, Linear Epidermal Nevus, Linear IgA Dermatosis (LAD), Lipodermatosclerosis, Lymphangioma Circumscriptum, Miliaria, Molluscum Contagiosum, Neurofibromatosis, Nickel Dermatitis, Onychomadesis, Onychomycosis, Palmoplantar Eccrine Hidradenitis, Papular Pruritic Eruption (PPE), Paronychia, Pellagra, Pemphigus Foliaceous,

Pemphigus Vulgaris, Piebaldism, Pityriasis Rosea, Pityriasis Rubra Pilaris, Plantar Hyperkeratosis, Plantar Warts, Poikiloderma, Postinflammatory Hyperpigmentation and Hypopigmentation, Post Topical Steroids Hypopigmentation, Psoriasis, Pyogenic Granuloma or Lobular Capillary Hemangioma, Scabies, Seborrheic Dermatitis, Steven Johnson Syndrome (SJS) and Toxic Epidermal Necrolysis (TEN),

Sunburn, Systemic Sclerosis, Tinea Capitis, Tinea Pedis, Tinea Versicolor, Traction Alopecia, Urticaria, Vasculitis, Vitiligo, and Xanthelasma.

*****

www.ingramcontent.com/pod-product-compliance
Lightning Source LLC
Chambersburg PA
CBHW070808290526
45795CB00002B/662